IF IT HURTS

"Don't Do That"

James Richard Pierrot

Pilegasus

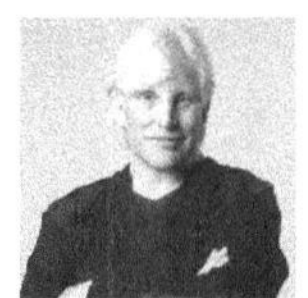

ISBN: 9798709370883
ASIN: B08WP375DM
Cover design by: Methodmike
Library of Congress Control Number: 2018675309
Printed in the United States of America

IF IT HURTS

"Don't Do That"

TABLE OF CONTENTS

Introduction
Commercials
The Science
Research
Opioid Use
Our Environment
Opioid Addiction
My Environment
Memory Lane
My Story
Prolong Narcotic Use
The Accident
No Re-Course
Resolved
Successful Recovery
Conclusion
Acknowledgement
Doing My Part
Disclaimer
The End

MR. JAMES RICHARD PIERROT

If It Hurts Don't Do That
Narcotic Free Pain Relief

INTRODUCTION

How is it, that there is so many book titles describing chronic cervical spine and back pain cures, but few who write about this subject have ever suffered or successfully defeated it for themselves. Certainly, they schill their agenda with the very treatments they're pushing, proclaiming they've used these devices on themselves as proof positive the gadget works.

COMMERCIALS

S hilling, especially on a television commercial will most always give the viewer a sense the presenter is a specialist. Their clients have the only miracle cure you need to resolve your pain.

We've all seen the accident commercials confirming the enormous settlements attorneys have received for their clients. They parade these very healthy-looking clients on screen proclaiming these attorneys have gotten them multi-million-dollar settlements, these are actors.

Radio is a bit more concealing and misleading, that's because you can't see the victim to whether the injury is genuine. If the actual persons stating this on TV were the client, having such a settlement, they'd be seen by viewers in a wheelchair, covered from head to toe in a body-cast.

Rarely if ever are these devices approved by a medical authority, or UL certified to ensure your safety. Commercials depend on a sense of gullibility to make the case you need to purchase these products. What you need to know with absolute certainty is, are these products sensible in their use, and are they sensible for you. The only sure way to know the safety issues as they apply to you,

and before you shell-out your hard-earned money, consult with your physician.

We've all googled or were at one time counselled by our physicians on the reasons we suffer pain. We all seem to cringe when our doctors, or insurance companies prescribe physical therapy either before surgery or after treatment.

Far too many patients who could benefit from the recovery success of physical therapy do not fully understand the steps in a healing process, nor what is necessary to successfully make a full-pain free recovery from invasive surgery. They instead toss their scripts before ever giving scar reduction, or strength training treatments the opportunity to shorten their recovery. Physical therapy performed in a controlled safe environment shortens recovery time dramatically.

Physical Therapy is absolutely needed when the surgeon through an incision invades your body. Muscles are often cut during such a procedure.

Patience not fully informed, have not had the need fully explained as to the benefits of physical therapy do not generally realize without those services their recovery is most often prolonged. The lack of knowledge, the risk potential is re-injuring the surgical area.

"If it hurts, don't do that". This is the best advice my therapist ever spewed my way.

THE SCIENCE

We've all learned while attending our grammar-school science studies, what makes up the content of the basic human anatomy. Within us there exists a skeletal-structure made up of vertebra, muscles, tendons, nerves, blood-vessels, the heart, a bag of sorts that's covered in a layer of skin that holds all this good stuff together. The main orchestrator and monitor of this entire miracle package: the brain. Nerves feed the brain; the brain responds by conducting the many components within our anatomy accordingly.

All our bodily parts in one way or another interconnect, connected in such a way that they must remain in harmony with one another to perform the work designed by the creator. Any one of them out of sync with the rest, mis-behaves in some odd way, we feel as discomfort and depending on the intensity of the discomfort, the sensation often is felt as pain.

RESEARCH

I f you're anything like me, you perform relentless due-diligent research and you quickly discovered how limited pain medication can be. All medications have side-effects, some-worse than others.

Those that cause bodily harm such as drugs containing "Nonsteroidal anti-inflammatories, technically referred to as an "NSAID". There use as pain relivers over a prolonged period of time can and often does cause a reduction in kidney function.

With extended use, drugs containing this ingredient can induce stage-three kidney-disease. Worse yet if used over a period of time will very likely cause full kidney failure, stage-five kidney-disease is likely the result. If stage-five kidney disease becomes your diagnosis, weekly dialysis visits will become an integral part of your busy agenda.

OPIOID USE

Limited Opioid use has its benefits, doesn't mess with your kidneys as NSAID's do. While this drug bypasses the kidneys, prolonged use causes addiction, and over time are less effective for limiting or even controlling your pain.

The risk of death with extended Opioid use is real, and without intervention you could find yourself as I certainly did, in a medical crisis battling its addictive side effects.

OUR ENVIRONMENT

The question most may have never asked of ourselves is how our environment, our behavior within our surroundings affects those nagging stimuli that encourage pain receptors to spontaneously drive us to our beds, incredibly nuts with agony. Some may even be driven to the not so unheard-of way out, suicide. It happens all too often, a painful chronic sensation that define our day as unworthy of the price to live it.

Pain isn't going to allow you to enjoy fun-filled activities when the discomfort controls' how we feel, how we interact with others, or why we're withdrawn to out of the way places.

OPIOID ADDICTION

We sit alone in the darkness because we can no longer tolerate an existence when chronic pain gets to be too much to bear. Our friends and families bear the brunt of our emotional stress. They tolerate knowing we do not feel well, often they don't understand our outbursts, nor why we have such an aggressive behavior when interacting with others while on Opioids.

Believe It or Not, Opioid Addicted is most likely your diagnosis. Intolerance and excessive stress are often clear evidence you're Opioid Addicted. This is the term social behavioral science uses to describe your odd behavior. It's time to seek medical help, your tolerance to the drug having taken it for far too long has awaken the monster within you.

The monster within you has no tolerance nor self-control, detoxing is the only option left to you, and most important, you can't do it by yourself. You need a physician's assistance to withdraw from its addictive effects safely. Detoxing off Opioids takes time, a reduction in the dosage you take until you can tolerate being without this medication.

Opioid addicted myself, I thought that I was dying, I was just that sick.

MY ENVIRONMENT

I'll asked this question again, it's that important. Have you ever asked yourself how my environment, my behavior, activities I pursue within it cause pain? Have you? This is the most important conversation you could ever have with yourself without being viewed psychotic by your family, friends, or colleagues.

MEMORY LANE

Before I answer this, Lets stroll down memory lane for an insight as to why I might know so very much more about this subject. More so than the specialists you've been feeding your hard-earned insurance dollars too for minimal relief.

Like many of us I researched endlessly in hopes of discovering a miracle cure that would give me some relief. All I wanted was physical security knowing I'd be okay, and a sense of well-being. With most there's always a gimmick, for example a specialized decompression machine promising permanent relief.

I have news for these folk's, "Permanent", doesn't mean shelling out another ninety-five to one-hundred-thirty-five dollars weekly for more of that miracle machines promise.

Decompression from these devices is most always temporary. For some, a good potential solution when the goal is to avoid surgery, but in the end the only long-term relief here with this device is continued use.

If you're recovering from frontal or posterior cervical spine or lower back surgery this is not a remedy for you. For some, these devices provide decompression relief, generally because their herniated disk hasn't fully degraded, and can in some instances be re-inflated over time.

This is a temporary pre-op treatment, should not be used as a post-op remedy for cervical pain without a physician's approval. An MRI, along with a doctor's approval, should be the only advice adhered to when considering decompression machines. There may be a great deal more going on along your spine you should have in-depth knowledge of, and before you engage treatment with decompression devices.

MY STORY

Cervical spine with low back pain. This is my success story living pain free without medication of any kind. I endured more than sixteen posterior procedures as well as frontal cervical spine operations over a course of twenty years. This did not include the two lower back procedures, nor the three vocal cord operations I underwent. Vocal cord alignment surgery was required to correct the damage caused by the many frontal procedures I endured. Separation of the vocal cords was due entirely to excessive scar tissue that led to a loss of vocal cord function and my ability to talk.

Mechanisms within the human body, those we depend on for our mobility have a skeletal structure with interlaced nerves, so many spider nerves winding their way through the many vertebra along our spines. Nerves transmit electrical pulses on their way to the brain. Compressed nerves reduce electrical flow, we feel a sensation of numbness. Significantly compressed, there can be a complete loss of sensation, and sensory function. Compressed further our mobility is often affected. Nerves are impinged when the spaces between the vertebra are adequately reduced to squeeze the nerve. What many books fail to talk about is how you can become pain free without kidney killing medications, while at the same time avoiding the risks of opioid addiction, and the use of hard narcotics for pain relief.

Medications are temporary remedies not intended to cure your pain but to ease it. How you live your life pain free can be accomplished by avoiding activities harmful to your mobility and to a complete recovery.

There are no quick fixes to cervical or lower back pain.

There is no miracle pain medication that provides long-lasting mind-boggling celebrated relief. All pain medications are temporary by design. They are not, at least none that I know of and I've taken them all, are intended for long term prolong use.

If limited use eliminated your pain, long term use would not be needed by design, you certainly wouldn't have to take two every few hours for relief.

There are side effects with all medications, prolonged use is a sure way of experiencing the many medication side effects labels warn against. Some even cause severe depression, a mental disorder driven by pain, chronic pain in some cases leads to the worse of outcomes, suicide.

We can live comfortably within our home and the spaces we occupy if we are in control of our environments and know our limitations.

THE ACCIDENT

An early evening trip home from work was interrupted as I waited to turn left onto a side street, my car rear-ended by another vehicle. An unintentional act for sure, the driver who hit me had been drinking. My car was totaled, the impact severe. I was struck from behind by the other vehicle doing 45 while I was stationary at a dead stop. The back of my driver's seat broke away, and I ended up in the rear seat. Ironically, I was wearing a seatbelt even then, no headrest to support my neck though. The seatbelt was of no help and I was seriously whiplashed. Mind-boggling numb while my car up on its side, I'd crawl out through the window after breaking the glass to exit the driver's door.

Years followed with significant pain I'd have to learn to live with. Back then cervical spine surgery was in its infancy, not yet a viable option to ease my pain. A neck brace was about all the relief doctors could provide. Headaches the worse imaginable would keep me in tears. I got through it for several years, while the pain seemed to ease as my tolerance to bear it heightened.

Some twenty years after that initial car accident I'd lose the use of my right arm while innocently sitting at my desk.

No pain to speak of, numb is all, still I lacked the strength and control to lift my arm. An MRI revealed the C4 vertebra had collapse, deteriorated over time with sharp ridges nearly severing the nerves running beneath. Obviously, surgery would be necessary to correct this, the c4 vertebra was broken.

This would be the first of many frontal procedures I'd endure. I regained full use of my right arm during recovery. Post-op recovery the bad news came, my doctor stated it's not over for you yet, more surgery soon would be needed.

Mis-diagnosed during recovery from my initial automobile accident led to the DE-genitive disc disease diagnosis that was now wearing away my spinal column. My doctor at the time, had no real case studies to rely on and he felt that I was faking the symptoms. A few years later C4 and C5 were fused with C6 to stabilize my cervical spine.

In February of 2001, while walking a top a grated floor, it collapsed beneath me. The jolt was so severe I hyperextended my neck backwards shattering every vertebra from C3 all the way through to T1. Ironically C4, C5, and C6 were strong enough to evade damage, but everything above and below was crushed. The pain just un-imaginable. The medical solution, a very long surgical procedure to place two steel frontal plates with four screws, accompanied by two steel rods posterior, boasting sixteen screws to hold this erector set all together. Robo-cop had more mobility than I, the pain was ungodly indescribable and for far too many years yet to come.

NO RE-COURSE

Permanently disabled, I'd learn to get by, few activities I could perform without suffering some sort of relapse, and another round of more of the same, pain. Heavily dependent on Opioids, I was taking as prescribed the maximum daily dosage followed by endless hours of sleep, I was emotionally a wreck. My life: hours of sleep not enough in the day to get beyond the intense pain. Awaken with pain, another dose of hard narcotics, within an hour I was right back in bed.

This went on for years. In 2011, I was so fed-up with pain, no life of any sorts to speak of. Doctors were not giving me more than a few years to live, I was horrified, scared to death for my young teenaged children. Told to get my affairs in order and to learn to live with it, by the many who could not and would not help me. I promise you if not for my young daughter I wanted so badly to toss the towel and let god take me. Severe pain, low self-esteem, it doesn't get any worse than this.

RESOLVED

I honestly had no clue Opioids were so unbelievably addictive until I decided to try living with the pain rather than spending my life in bed. I have never felt and been so sick. I was so incredibly ill, certain I would die. If not for my doctor realizing I had stopped taking my medication, dying wasn't all that a far-fetched reality, I was seriously sick.

Nearly a year would pass detoxing off the Opioids, before I'd begin to feel better, the pain wasn't as intolerable as it had once been.

Having been on Opioids for so long, my body never was able to adjust to the pain. The narcotics were deadening my pain whilst my body was deprived of the opportunity to adapt, to recover without their use.

A much younger me, I'd hung out at the local gym lifting weights to strengthen my back. There were always people walking around in fancy bodybuilding gear looking dapper in their sported outfits. The dudes sporting the muscles though were covered from head to toe, towels wrapped around their necks to keep their muscles warm. I took pointers from these guys, we talked about muscle burn and why I hurt so much.

Thinking back, I started looking into some of the things I

once did while bodybuilding to relieve muscle burn, knowing the burn came from tearing the muscle fiber.

Muscle burn is caused when muscle secrete an acid as it's worked. Body builders use Branch Chain Amino Acids, BCA's to neutralize the burning effect. In addition, BCA's support muscle healing with essential vitamins. I started again taking these and noticed within a few days I felt some relief, less pain when I moved around.

Scar tissue for me was a major issue and I had truckloads of it in my upper and lower back. Muscles not used weaken, spasm easily, more of an effort to do work is required then if the muscle were strong and flexible. When muscles harden along a scar line, a flexed muscle pulls against that scar tissue causing pain.

To limit the burning sensation I felt, whenever I was active, due entirely to having so much scar tissue along the surgical incision, I started massage therapy to reduce it. With deep penetrating massage, along with ultrasound treatments, I started to feel much better. Therapist's would explain keeping the muscle warm would help keep it flexible while the deep penetrating massage with ultrasound reduced the scar tissue by loosening and breaking up the scar tissue surrounding muscle fiber.

Keeping your injury warm, not hot, but at a comfortable temperature goes a long way to easing muscle soreness especially after surgery.

Excessive radiant heat directly on the injury, has the tendency to aggravate the area, inducing a spasm that pulls against the

injury, more pain is usually the result. Same can be said for excessive cold, the muscles contract, pulling against the scar tissue along the incision, again causing pain.

I've noticed numerous times patients in the doctor's office post-op wearing flimsy blouses, nothing covering their incisions, the hair standing up on the back of their necks from the cold produced by the air conditioning. They were complaining how much pain they were in, all along not having a clue their discomfort along with increased sensitivity was self-induced.

The muscles along the injury, chilled by the AC would spasm, pulling against the wound. It seemed looking good while miserably in pain, was significantly more important than keeping the injured area warm.

Keeping the incision comfortably warm really is a big deal when you're recovering from surgical pain. The incision area maintained at a comfortable temperature is a must, along with weekly massage therapy to reduce scar tissue keeps the muscles from hardening. This is key to achieving a life pain free after any type of back or cervical spine surgery.

Ten days is all anyone should be given narcotics for surgical pain. Knowing what causes the pain after you stop the narcotics is how you'll recover more efficiently and completely.

Remaining covered up, your body will adjust to your sur-

roundings. Afterall being stripped down in theheat doesn't keep you cool. If it did, camel jockeys in the desert would not be fully covered up during the hottest time of the day. Wearing lightly colored clothing in the direct sun deflects the suns radiant heat. While wearing warm clothing to avoid direct cold. Our bodies adapt to our surroundings, if the environment we exist in is affecting us uncomfortably, it may very well be necessary to take life changing steps for our bodies to heal efficiently.

So often we tend to continue our lifestyles long after we've undergone a significant surgical procedure. Not realizing you may no longer be able to continue living your life as you once did.

If it hurts don't do that, it's not just nonsense rhetoric. Pain is a signal something isn't right, adjusting your lifestyle accordingly to accommodate it may make the most sense.

During my recovery, I was considered permanently disabled, I did not sit around feeling sorry for myself. Instead I went back to college, I did so because I was no longer able to do those things I once did.

Not able to do them wasn't the end of my life, I needed to adapt and learned to enjoy those things I could still do comfortably. Ironically, I became much happier with my new job opportunities, then I ever was in my previous. Yes, that's correct, I am no longer disabled. I live entirely pain free taking not one pill of any kind for pain relief. Occasionally I'll head back to my therapist for a nice massage, but no longer do I do it for pain relief.

Reducing pain through physical therapy to minimize scar tissue, while remaining covered up keeping your injury a comfortable temperature goes a long way to support healing.

Staying out of direct sunlight, avoiding excessive hot or cold temperatures on your injury will make your life a whole lot happier.

Medicine is constantly evolving; new tools are available to surgeons today reducing the surgical recovery time. My mobility has been restored near ninety-five percent. Peak fusion cages, along with D-trac devices, all played a huge role in restoring my mobility. No longer is my cervical spine supported with steel plates, contoured rods, and a vast assortment of titanium screws.

To live a life pain free, to fully recover from any kind of surgical procedure, its essential you take care of the area operated on. Any muscle cut regardless of how, it takes time and care to fully heal.

Successful Recovery

- Understand all facets of your medical procedure, ask all the questions you need answers too, and ask as many times as you need too, to feel comfortable in your decision to move forward with a surgical procedure.
- Know-how your daily activities will affect your recovery after surgery and adjust them accordingly.
- Pre-plan, then arrange for the care you'll need post-op, decide how and whom will administer your post-op plan. This should include physical therapy, scar tissue remediation as well as muscle strengthening exercises.
- Pre-planning steps reduces the stress you'll most likely be unable to deal with for the first few days post-op. While prior arrangements for your care helps obtain the support you need without delay.
- Follow through with your post-op plan, heeding your doctor's advice. While obtaining the medical assistance needed pre-op and prescribed by your doctor, ensures it's available when you need those services.
- Reduce your need for narcotics gradually minimizing any potential withdrawal symptoms.
- Understand what pain medications are best for you, know which of them have harmful side effects then limit how often you take them.
- Have all medications prescribed on-hand before you undergo your procedure.
- Give your body its natural ability, and time needed to heal on its terms.
- Adapt to your environment by addressing your

surgical-site exposure to the elements. Keep the surgical site comfortably warm by adjusting your clothing for conditions to avoid muscles spasms.

- If muscle spasms occur, relax, address the spasm with comfortable clothing. Adjust your body temperature for comfort, create a surrounding that encourages a relaxing calm, then take deep cleansing breaths to reduce muscle stress.
- With your doctor's approval, consider joining a fitness club. Take full advantage of the club's exercise equipment. Most definitely take advantage of the waterjet massage beds many have. Waterjet beds do wonders to control physical stress, they massage, and they are significantly less expensive resources than medical services.

CONCLUSION

Pre-planned steps, arranging for all your support needs prior to your procedure will help you quickly address any surgical stress post-op.

Knowing there is a process in place, pre-planning will help you deal with your recovery, reducing the stress you'll inevitably find yourself coping with afterwards.

ACKNOWLEDGEMENT

There is no greater statement that I can make than to acknowledge the great works of all the wonderful men and women who gave of themselves to help me through some of the most difficult times in my life.

In September of 2008, I stood before Dr. Jeffery Lewis, a cane in hand to steady myself, head hung forward unsupported off to one side, I was completely unable to lift it. Arms motionless hanging to my sides as well, I could not raise them but a few inches.

I literally had no ability to walk more than a few feet unassisted, and it was painfully obvious I was in severe distress, I needed help and Dr. Lewis was prepared to give it.

Dr. Lewis explored the many options for a surgical procedure to regain some sense of comfort. Not one discouraging word as others had expressed that he could not or would not help me.

Dr. Lewis exhibited a sense of control, a professionalism I had not seen in others. He spoke very little; exhibited an immense sense of confidence in himself and his team's abilities to bring to a successful conclusion this surgical procedure that so many before he had said could not be accomplished without ending in my death.

No pain, no gain is not just a manta of wisdom, nor is it nonsense rhetoric. It's a fact when your life hangs in the balance. The pain was immense, but the reward when it was all said and done was so very much worth all I had suffered. Dr. Lewis not only returned all my physical functions, but I regained full mobility. I am significantly better today than I have been in a very long time. I was back on track living my life pain free, and very grateful for all Dr. Lewis and his staff had done for me.

DOING MY PART

My surgical procedure was behind me but not the end of my journey to a full recovery. Taking the next step in my pre-planning, following through doing my part post-op with the care I needed. Minimizing the use of the narcotics prescribed to just a few days started me down a path to recovery.

By reducing my narcotic intake for pain post-op, I'd avoid addiction withdrawal symptoms giving my body the opportunity to adapt naturally. Medication for mild pain most often is not necessary, instead choose one of the therapy practices learned as an alternate to narcotic pills. If medication is needed for intolerance, take an over the counter non-NSAID, like Tylenol, you'll be avoiding the risk of stage-three kidney disease for prolonged use.

Keeping appointments with a physical therapist for the full duration of your needed treatment will keep scar tissue from forming to a minimum. Reducing scar tissue, and keeping the muscles flexible, will immensely alleviate muscle spasm pain associated with surgery. Soreness is not the same as pain, in time even that will completely resolve. As the muscles heal, and the nerves regenerate, the spasms subside as well.

Standing in your doctor's office, screaming at the top of

your lungs proclaiming how much pain you're in, isn't helping you, nor is it doing much for those sharing the waiting room.

Over time I have watched so many patients do exactly this, and all along blaming their doctors for their discomfort they took no responsibility for themselves.

Dis-comfort more often than not, the patient has control over. Taking responsibility for yourself is step one, owning it, then following a well thought out recovery plan. Surgery is most certainly painful, no one is denying that. Doctors open your trunk and rearrange the items to help you get back on your feet. This is the first step, steps two, three, right on through to twenty-five are yours alone to take with your doctor's assistance.

You must do your part; you can help yourself by helping your body adapt naturally. Know how the pain medications you're taking delays your recovery time. Know how it prolongs your body's natural abilities to adapt, to heal, and minimize its use.

Cover up, address your environmental needs, and adapt to your surgical condition. You're not just a buck ninety-eight collection of chemicals, you have the ability to adapt, to change, and to become more than you ever thought possible.

THE END

DISCLAIMER

The author does not claim any professional expertise nor are any expressed. The author's knowledge is expressed as personal knowledge and is based on his experiences with chronic cervical spine, neck and back pain. Always seek the advice of a trained professional before attempting anything expressed herein.

ACKNOWLEDGEMENT

To Dr. Jeffery Lewis and his entire staff, you have my deepest graditude for all you've done for me.